A Lifetime of Beauty

The Definitive All-Natural Guide to Skin and Hair Care

By
Joni Loughran

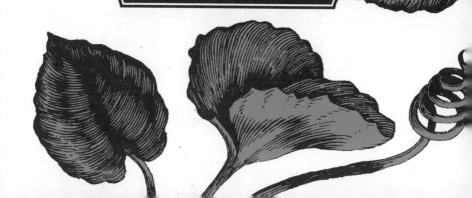

A LIFETIME OF BEAUTY

THE DEFINITIVE
ALL-NATURAL GUIDE TO
SKIN AND HAIR CARE

Cover Design and Graphics by: Blackburn Design

Published by:

Summerflight Publishing
P.O. Box 751261
Petaluma, CA 94975

DEDICATION

To my clients: you have been my best teachers.

AUTHOR'S NOTE

I have been working with clients, friends, and family using an 'as close to nature as possible' approach for twenty years. When I began, I was drawn to this philosophy as if there were no alternatives. As the years have passed, I feel only stronger about this conviction.

My attraction to the gifts and strengths of nature was nurtured by my father's love of plants and his religious beliefs to live close to God (God and nature go hand in hand). I was influenced by people who I admired – they had a certain affinity to, and respect for, nature. However, nothing has been more affirming to me that the 'natural' approach is right than working with people on a one-to-one basis – watching their complexion improve and become vibrant, watching their hair become shiny and beautiful – this is positive confirmation that 'natural' works!

Though the intent of my practice is to watch my clients' complexions and hair become more beautiful, an interesting transformation inevitably takes place. Those who are dedicated to improving their skin and hair also experience a greater sense of well-being. In many cases, their health improves, for, in the end, in order to have beautiful skin and hair – you need to take care of yourself. Perhaps vanity is the best excuse to live a more healthy lifestyle.

There is one last impression that working with natural methods and natural cosmetics has made on me. People do better – physically, emotionally, and spiritually – when they maintain a 'connectedness' with nature. Human beings become lost when they no longer see the green of a forest, feel the grass beneath their feet, or smell a true floral fragrance. They lose peace. This association with nature needs to be maintained and fostered. As subtle as it may be, using natural cosmetics that are laden with essential oils, herbal extracts, and the cold-pressed oils of fruits and vegetables – applying them to your skin – is one way to maintain this connection. And though it may be subtle, it is powerful.

INTRODUCTION

My professional niche as a skin care specialist (aesthetician) and cosmetologist is to work closely with nature and the nature of human beings. My practice is based on this philosophy. In my work with clients, this translates into using cosmetics that contain the highest quality natural ingredients and using alternative, natural therapies such as hydrotherapy, acupressure, massage, and aromatherapy to de-stress the client and nurture the skin and hair.

The goal of my first appointment with a client is to design an individualized program that will improve the complexion and the condition of her hair as well as guide her in product selection. This program is based on the principles listed in "A Checklist for Beautiful Skin" and "The Basics of Natural Hair Care." In addition, I want each client to understand the reasons behind the design of her program. In the past, I have provided many handouts and articles for my clients to read, but there was a need to consolidate this information and make it easily available. That is the reason I have written this book.

This book is divided into the three important areas of personal care: skin care, hair care, and make-up. The skin care section provides guidelines to determine skin 'type' and how the skin should be cleansed, toned, and moisturized. Effective, special treatments such as exfoliating, steaming, facial misting, and the use of masks can be incorporated to enhance the basic skin care program. Because skin care does not stop at the neck, "Skin Care for the Body" describes how to give care and attention to the rest of your body. "The Basics of Natural Hair Care" offers a five-step program to attaining a shiny, attractive head of hair and discusses the practices that will prevent hair damage.

The final section, "The Basics of Make-up Artistry and Using Naturally Pigmented Cosmetics," is an adjunct to skin care. It is an important section because most women use make-up and though they want to take good care of their skin, they often neglect to scrutinize their make-up. Included are guidelines for color application and the reasons to use naturally pigmented cosmetics. Together, these three sections will guide the reader to enjoy a lifetime of beautiful skin and hair.

TABLE OF CONTENTS

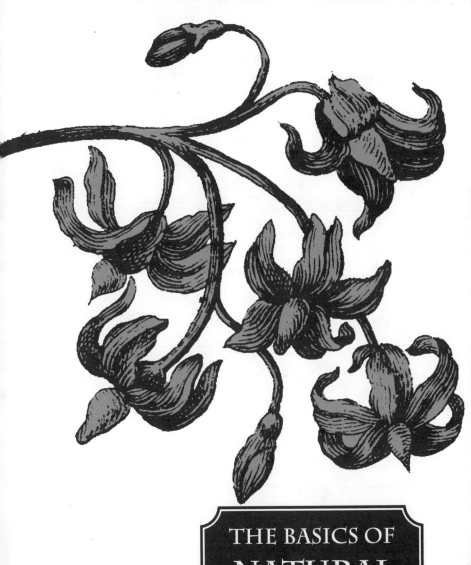

THE BASICS OF
NATURAL
SKIN CARE

A CHECKLIST FOR BEAUTIFUL SKIN

*N*atural skin care is both an art and a science. It encompasses everything that has an influence on the skin's condition and appearance. It requires getting to know your skin and paying close attention to what the skin is communicating and how it may be changing. It also requires, as a foundation, an understanding of the skin's many functions and how those functions can be nurtured.

A person's skin covers an average of nineteen square feet and weighs about seven pounds. A cross section reveals three defined layers. The *epidermis* is the outermost layer, known as the cuticle or protective layer, and is made of tightly packed, scale-like cells which are continually being shed. An entirely new cuticle layer of skin forms approximately every twenty-eight days. (This is believed to slow down with age.) The next layer is the *dermis*. It is also called the 'true skin' because most of the vital functions of the skin are performed or housed here. It contains the glands that secrete perspiration and sebum (oil), the papilla (hair manufacturing plant), nerve fibers, blood vessels, lymph glands, and sense receptors. The dermis has an elastic quality that is due to the protein connective tissues called elastin and collagen. Together, they allow for strength, resiliency, and flexibility. Below the dermis is the third layer, called the *subcutaneous* layer. It is made of a fatty tissue that gives the body smoothness and contour and serves as a shock absorber for the vital organs. In addition, it stores energy and is an effective insulator. Together, these three layers form the miraculous 'living fabric' known as skin.

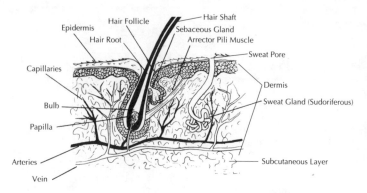

The skin serves to maintain our health and well-being in an amazing variety of ways. In one square centimeter (the size of your fingertip), there are one hundred sweat glands, twelve feet of nerves, hundreds of nerve endings, ten hair follicles, twenty sebaceous glands, six feet of blood vessels, sixteen heat sensors, four cold sensors, and thousands of cells. Unbroken, the skin is our first line of defense against disease and bacterial invasion. It regulates body temperatures, sends neurological messages to the brain, detoxifies by excreting wastes from the body, respirates (absorbs oxygen and releases carbon dioxide), absorbs nutrients, manufactures vitamin D, and protects the body from ultra violet damage from the sun.

Natural skin care recognizes that the skin is our largest vital organ and that it requires care and attention to look its best and to maintain peak performance. Factors that influence its condition are either internal or external. As you read through this checklist, ask yourself, "How well am I taking care of my skin? How well am I doing in this particular area?" Evaluate. Armed with this information, you can take better care of your skin and, ultimately, better care of yourself. If these factors are considered and practiced, you can look forward to a lifetime of beautiful skin.

#1
STAY OUT OF THE SUN!

$\mathcal{P}$eter Pugliese, M.D., a biomedical researcher who has been studying the skin's response to sunlight, states that 90% of the skin problems associated with ageing are the result of too much exposure to the sun. These symptoms include premature wrinkling; dry, leathery skin; sagging skin; distended capillaries; blotchy pigmentation; and skin cancer.

Vanity is one concern, and health is another. Ninety percent of all skin cancers develop on sun-exposed areas of the body. Skin cancer is increasing at an alarming rate in the United States and will claim between 7,000 and 8,000 lives this year. Dermatologists say those who are at high risk are people with fair skin, blond or red hair, blue or green eyes, sun sensitivity, freckles, large or numerous moles, a family history of melanoma, and any people who have suffered from a blistering sunburn anytime in their lives. The Skin Cancer Foundation recommends starting sun protection in childhood, as soon as children go out in the sun. Researchers feel that if a Sun Protection Factor (SPF) 15 is used during the first eighteen years of life, skin cancer can be reduced by 78%. However, even when wearing a sunblock, people need to limit their exposure to the sun, especially high-risk people.

Guidelines for preventing the sun-damage symptoms of ageing and skin cancer are:

- Stay out of the sun as much as possible.

- In particular, avoid extensive sun exposure between 10am and 3pm, even if wearing a sunblock.

- Beware of reflected light from sand, water, cement, and snow.

- Wear a sunscreen that provides both UVA and UVB protection with an SPF of at least 15.

- Apply sunscreen 30 minutes before going out in the sun and re-apply it every hour when swimming or perspiring. Don't forget to protect your lips and the tops of your ears – they are often forgotten and are just as much at risk.

- For extra protection, use clothing such as long sleeved shirts, long-legged pants, and a sun hat. Sunglasses will help for around the eyes.

- Avoid tanning booths and sunlamps.

- If you spend a great deal of time in the sun, have your skin thoroughly checked by a dermatologist once a year, especially if you have a number of moles.

#2
DON'T SMOKE!

Cigarette smoking robs the skin of its vitality and its potential for being smooth and attractive. There are approximately 4,000 chemical compounds that are produced when tobacco burns. Among those considered harmful are acetone, ammonia, arsenic, benzene, carbon monoxide, formaldehyde, hydrogen cyanide, and nicotine. The skin particularly suffers from smoking due to the harmful effects of carbon monoxide and nicotine on the circulatory system, depriving the skin tissue of much-needed oxygen and vital nutrients.

People who smoke have a depleted, pallid (almost grey) complexion that wrinkles prematurely. In addition, this type of skin does not heal well or rejuvenate quickly. If fact, it is not uncommon for plastic surgeons to refuse to perform cosmetic surgery on people who smoke because of the likelihood of slow, unsuccessful healing.

Another cosmetic consequence of smoking was discovered by researchers at the Medical College of Wisconsin. It seems that women who smoke one pack of cigarettes a day or more have a 50% greater chance of developing facial hair. It is speculated that this is caused by the effect smoking has on the ovaries and/or hormonal metabolism.

Although these cosmetic reasons for avoiding smoking may appeal to your vanity, smoking's real curse is to your overall health. Smoking is the largest single cause of preventable death. Lung diseases such as cancer, emphysema, or bronchitis can result. The lungs are damaged by smoking, and their natural cleansing process is crippled. If you smoke one pack a day, in a year you have will poured one cup of tar into your lungs, tar that is rich in cancer-producing chemicals. The air passageways in the lungs become irritated and produce excess mucous which provides a breeding ground for bacteria and viruses. Smoking is considered to be a leading cause of coronary artery disease. It damages the lining of the arteries, encouraging plaque formation, which narrows the artery walls. The nicotine makes the heart beat faster and require more oxygen, but the carbon monoxide decreases the amount of oxygen the blood can carry. This has an adverse effect on the cardiovascular system. Smoking has also been linked to blood disease, ulcers, and a decline in immune function. Smoking worsens virtually every health condition or disease. The best advice: if you don't smoke, don't start; if you <u>do</u> smoke, quit!

#3
EXERCISE!

*P*eople who are physically fit both look and feel good. A regular aerobic work out combined with flexibility and strength exercises will keep a person in top physical shape. This kind of conditioning will lengthen your life, improve your appearance, build your self-confidence, reshape your figure, and delay the ageing process.

Exercise benefits the skin and aids in maintaining a clear, youthful complexion by increasing circulation, calming the nerves, and promoting a deeper, more revitalizing sleep. Even the best skin care program will not be as effective without regular exercise.

#4
GET ENOUGH REST
AND RELAXATION!

*P*eople lead very busy lives today, juggling jobs and families. We seem to be on the go from morning until night. In addition, we know that we need to exercise to stay fit. All of this activity needs to be balanced with enough rest, relaxation, and sleep.

Sleep scientists and researchers feel that sleepiness has become an epidemic in this country and contributes to chronic fatigue, poor work production, ill humor, and dissatisfaction with life. It is also a leading cause of car accidents.

How do you know if you are getting enough sleep? Dr. Wilse Webb, a sleep research pioneer, says if you have to wake up to an alarm, "you are shortening your natural sleep pattern." To correct it, you must go to bed early enough that you wake up on your own at the time you want to arise.

When you are well rested, rejuvenated, and getting enough sleep, your skin will mirror this vitality with a healthful glow.

#5
LIMIT YOUR ALCOHOL!

*R*ecent studies are now showing that alcohol consumption for even moderate drinkers (one to two ounces per day) can lead to damaged livers and a variety of cancers and may contribute to osteoporosis and depression. Anything that has this kind of effect on your general health is going to affect the skin.

Alcohol dehydrates the skin and impedes circulation, thus robbing it of precious moisture and vital nutrients. It can lead to broken or distended capillaries, especially over the nose and cheeks. It also depletes the body of vitamins and minerals needed for a healthy complexion. Recent studies have shown that <u>women</u> are more susceptible to the ill effects of alcohol than are men. Because women are generally more concerned about their appearance, it would be prudent to reduce or eliminate alcohol intake.

#6
COSMETICS...
USE ONLY THE BEST!

A skin care program is put together with three cosmetics....a cleanser, a toner, and a moisturizer. An expanded program will include an eye cream or oil, a mask, and an exfoliant. Because the cosmetics are the cornerstone of every skin care program, the quality of the program depends on the quality of the cosmetics. Cosmetics with inferior ingredients can actually harm the skin by drying it out, irritating it, or blocking the pores.

Using poor quality cosmetics may be worse than using nothing at all. In my practice, I have seen women of all ages and all walks of life. Many times, those who did very little to their skin had better looking skin than women who had experimented with every sort of commercial product that was new on the market – often times loaded with artificial ingredients – be it scrubs, soaps, or creams.

What makes high quality cosmetics? First, read the

ingredients on the label of the product. The unfamiliar words can be confusing, so you will need to arm yourself with a book about cosmetic ingredients (e.g., The Consumer's Dictionary of Cosmetic Ingredients by Ruth Winter). The best cosmetics will read like a food label, with easily recognizable ingredients. Surprisingly, however, you will find that some of those long, strange-looking ingredients are from natural sources and just fine for use. Next, investigate the integrity of the manufacturer and the manufacturing process. What are the company's standards? How long has it been in business? Does it have a philosophy that appeals to you? Is it using quality raw ingredients that have value in cosmetics? Does it support its products with dependable customer service? Many times, these questions can be answered by salespeople, but ask more than one to be sure the information you get is consistent. You can also contact the manufacturer directly.

When you have set your criteria and are satisfied with the outcome of your investigation, you should test the product to see how you react to it. An experienced salesperson or aesthetician can recommend a line of skin care products, but no one will be able to tell you unequivocally what will work the best for you. That will only be known from the experience of using it.

The finest products for the best prices are available in natural/health food stores. This is not to say that they are all good...you will still need to read the labels. However, there is a wide variety of products at a variety of prices, and your chances are very good for finding a product with which you will be happy.

#7

BREATHE WELL!

*O*xygen is our most vital nutrient. We can live for weeks without food and days without water but only a few minutes without oxygen. The art and influence of the breath has been a part of religious, philosophical, and health disciplines through the ages. The breath is life itself.

Most people think that breathing correctly is a natural instinct. Certainly, we all breathe, but it is the quality of breathing that makes the difference, and it affects the quality of our lives and is reflected in the quality of our complexion.

A very simple deep-breathing exercise is to lie on your back and slowly fill with air, your abdomen, then the stomach, the lower lung, and lastly, the upper lung. To exhale, empty the abdomen first, then the stomach, and then the lungs. On the exhale, pause for a moment before you inhale again. (This technique was taught to me by a yoga instructor.)

Learning to breathe consciously can bring about clearer thinking, increased circulation, positive changes in moods and emotions, stress reduction, and more energy...resulting in a more beautiful complexion.

#8

DRINK PLENTY OF WATER!

*T*he role that water plays in our body is very interesting. More than half of our body weight is water. It is the basis of all body fluids, including perspiration, blood, lymph, urine, and digestive juices. Water helps to regulate our body temperature and is essential to keep food moving through the intestinal tract. It is also a lubricant throughout the body for joints and mucous membranes.

For our skin, water is essential for hydration to keep our skin moist, supple, and clear. Think of it as moisturizing your skin from the inside out. Lack of moisture is one of the main causes of wrinkles. Drinking two to three pints of clean, pure water a day is recommended for the average person. However, hot weather and exercising require an increase in this amount. (Sodas, coffee, teas, juices, and alcohol do not count.)

In addition to skin hydration, there are other benefits from drinking plenty of water. It is a natural appetite suppressant and is therefore an essential part of a weight loss program. It also maintains muscle and skin tone, and it rids the body of waste materials.

#9

EAT ONLY THE BEST FOODS!

*T*he physical human body was designed to be nourished from the plants and animals from the earth, in their natural form. This was true at the appearance of modern man nearly 40,000 years ago and remains true today because physiologically, we have not changed that much.

Considering individual needs (which will vary depending on body size, gender, health, exposure to pollutants, amount of exercise, and age), eating a varied diet that is rich in whole, natural foods, balanced in protein, fats, and carbohydrates, and void of chemicals, adulteration, and refinement will allow humans to realize their potential as physical, intellectual, emotional, and spiritual beings. Certainly the health and beauty of the skin depends on a balanced, natural diet. (The best foods, the best supplements, and the best information about healthy eating are found in natural/health food stores.)

In addition to this complete, natural diet, the skin needs a diet that includes plenty of liquids (for hydration), essential fatty acids (for suppleness, smoothness, and softness), and anti-oxidants (to inhibit free radical damage and slow the visible signs of ageing).

You may also consider the possibility of vitamin supplementation. A vitamin and mineral program may be warranted. Because of our biochemical individuality, such a program will be different for everyone, and you may want to see a nutritionist to get you on the right track.

If you are experiencing any unexplained health problems, it is highly recommended that you get tested for food allergies and/or hidden food allergies. You may be eating the very best of natural foods but if you are overly sensitive (allergic) to them, you will not look or feel your best. Allergic reactions can take a variety of forms such as fatigue, headaches, digestive problems, mood swings, skin problems, and weakened immune function. (For more information about testing for food allergies, call Immuno Lab, 1-800-231-9197).

#10

STRESS!

*T*here are different types of stress: mental, emotional, and physical. Of these, emotional stress tends to take the greatest toll on people. Stress is not all bad; in fact, life really would not be very interesting if we were not met with challenges. However, too much stress, too often with no effective and appropriate outlet, does not allow the body and soul to recuperate. As a result, our health as well as our complexion can suffer. Because we cannot change the events in our lives (and isn't life full of surprises?), we must learn to change our attitude and shore up our abilities to cope. Meditation, creative visualization, counseling, proper breathing, massage, regular exercise, getting more sleep, improving the diet, and spiritual pursuits have all helped people deal with stress. One thing that is nice to remember is that everyone's life is stressful at one time or another. It is a shared human experience.

DETERMINING YOUR SKIN TYPE

*P*hysiologically speaking, everyone's skin is the same, serving as one's largest vital organ. Yet, there are differences in characteristics that are the result of heredity, lifestyle, or the passage of time that classify skin as a certain 'type.' Knowing your skin 'type' will enable you to correctly select cosmetic preparations and use guidelines by which to treat your skin so that it will look its best.

NORMAL SKIN

Many people between the ages of twenty to thirty-five will fall into this category (although there are always exceptions). Normal skin indicates that the water and oil glands on the face are producing just the right amount to hydrate and protect the skin. The appearance of the skin is moist and dewy. The pores are small to medium in size. There are few or no blemishes. It is of medium thickness and has an even tone. Normal skin is smooth and firm with good elasticity. It may have some oiliness in the "T zone" (the forehead, nose, and chin), but unless the oil is excessive, the skin is still considered normal.

OILY SKIN

In oily skin, the sebaceous glands are producing too much oil. The pores are medium to large in size, and the skin has a shiny appearance. Oily skin is usually thicker and less sensitive than the other types. It appears most often in ages twelve to twenty-two, but some people may have oily skin all of their lives – gradually becoming less oily as they age. Although there is a tendency for clogged pores, blackheads, and blemishes, the good news is that oily skin does not show the signs of ageing as quickly.

DRY SKIN

Dry skin can be lacking in either oil or water or both. Skin that lacks water is called dehydrated skin. If the skin is thin and the pores are barely visible, it is lacking in oil (and possibly water as well). If the skin is thick with visible pores but has the characteristics of dry skin, it is probably only lacking water (usually the result of a poor skin care program).

Many people think that they have dry skin when they actually have superficial dryness. Superficial dryness is caused by the environment (sun, sea air, wind, pollutants) and improper skin care habits. A well-designed skin care program can eliminate the causes of superficial dryness.

Dry skin can be seen in people of all ages. Dry skin can feel tight and may have visible flaking, and it may be delicate and easily irritated. Signs of ageing, such as lines and creases, will appear sooner in this type of skin than the others. It has a matte finish with no sheen and sometimes has a rough feel to it.

COMBINATION SKIN

Combination skin is oily in certain areas and then dry or normal in the other areas. The most common combination skin is dryness in the cheeks and around the eyes with oiliness in the "T-zone" (the forehead, nose, and chin).

Combination skin is considered to be the most common of all the skin types and can be seen in people of all ages but most typically in people ages twelve to forty-five.

SENSITIVE SKIN

The dictionary defines sensitive as "readily or excessively affected by external influences." That, indeed, describes sensitive skin. It is easily irritated by the environment, harsh cosmetics, and rough treatment. Care must be taken to avoid products that contain alcohol, artificial colors, artificial fragrances, and highly active ingredients (which, unfortunately, may include essential oils and herbal extracts). Preservatives can also cause problems. There is a tendency with sensitive skin to have distended (broken) capillaries and allergies, and it usually sunburns very easily. This condition can be present in normal, dry, and oily skins and at any age.

ACNEIC SKIN

This type of skin is most common during the teenage years when hormones play havoc with our minds and bodies (stimulating the sebaceous glands), but it is not uncommon to find examples of 'adult acne.' 'Adult acne' is often the result of a change in health, the use of poor cosmetics, or cosmetic allergies. Acneic skin is characterized by chronic pustules, blackheads, and whiteheads. Unfortunately, this condition often causes scarring. There are varying degrees of 'problem' skin, and not all skin that is having trouble with blemishes can truly be called acneic. However, at any degree it is a most unwanted, unfortunate condition.

It is important for people with acne to realize that acne is not a normal condition. It is a symptom of a physical imbalance that may be different in each person who is afflicted. Because of this, there is no _one_ cure for acne. An acneic condition may stem from a deep-rooted systemic imbalance, a superficial systemic problem, or external causes. The dermatologist's only weapon is drug therapy, which is not a healthy solution but may be the only course that someone in a desperate situation can take. Natural methods – an integrated program of correct skin care, skin care products, diet, and lifestyle habits – _can_ be successful, but it takes time, dedication, and discipline. Guidance from naturopathic physicians, nutritionists, and skin care professionals can be of great help.

AGEING SKIN

Ageing is an additional characteristic that may be combined with any of the other skin types. The condition of the skin may be appropriate for the age of the individual, or it may be 'premature.' Appropriate ageing is the result of the passage of time and the slowing down of the glandular functions in the skin and its ability to rejuvenate. Premature ageing can be the result of overexposure to the sun (the number one cause), smoking, improper skin care, mistreatment, poor lifestyle habits, or health problems. It means that the skin looks older than it should.

Visible signs of ageing begin developing by the age of thirty, though for some they will show sooner and for others, later. Lines, wrinkles, dryness, roughness, and sagging are the most common signs of ageing skin.

DETERMINING YOUR SKIN TYPE

Before deciding to which 'type' you belong, also consider your heritage. Different atmospheres and weather conditions exist all over the world. Generally, extreme climates – both hot and cold – produce thicker-skinned people. Hot climates produce people with more color and more oil in the skin. People from moist, cool climates usually have thin, dry, sensitive skin. Where did your ancestors come from? This is a clue to your skin type.

After reading the descriptions and acknowledging your heritage, use your sight and your touch to make a final analysis.

This accounting should be done in the morning. The evening before, wash and rinse your face thoroughly with a very mild soap (this _one_ time only!). Do not apply any moisturizer or night creams. Upon arising, take a sheet of tissue paper and hold it against your face. Then, examine the tissue paper. Are there oil marks on it? In what areas? Take a close look at your skin in the mirror with natural light. What do the pores look like? Is the skin shiny or dull in appearance? Correlate this information with the descriptions of the basic skin types.

Next, use your sense of touch. Does the skin feel rough or tight? Does it have an oily feel to it? In which areas? Make a note of your findings.

After you have done this, rinse your face with warm water and pat it dry. It is best if you can take a second and third accounting of the skin during the day. Do not apply any moisturizer or make-up. A few hours after the first checking, examine your skin again with sight and touch. Rinse and pat dry, and then check one more time a few hours later. This type of analysis will give you a good idea of how much and where your skin is producing oil.

Once you have determined your skin type, keep in mind that the skin is in a state of transition and can change. This means that periodically you will need to re-evaluate your skin. This transition might be the result of your skin care program, the environment, your diet, general health, stress, or the ageing process. Although you may have normal skin today, after years pass, it may become dry. It is not uncommon for people with oily skin in their youth to develop normal skin as they age. Damaged and superficially dry skin can recapture its vitality with proper care. You may even notice a difference in your skin with the turn of the seasons. These changes in the skin need to be recognized as they will determine its immediate condition and will effect the design of your current skin care program.

THE BASICS: CLEANSING, TONING, MOISTURIZING

*A*fter you have determined your skin type, the next step is to put together your skin care program. You will need to determine what types of products to use, the techniques of their use, and the routine with which you will use them. The basics of every skin care routine are cleansing, toning, and moisturizing. (For guidelines in selecting your products, see #6 in "A Checklist For Beautiful Skin.") The goal is to have clean, toned, protected skin that is nourished and nurtured so that it will look its best!

CLEANSERS

Your natural skin care program begins with proper cleansing to remove make-up, accumulated dirt, the waste products excreted by the skin, and dead skin cells. If this process is done correctly, it helps prevent problems that can be caused by these factors, such as clogged pores, skin irritations or blemishes, and premature ageing. There are two rules of thumb for cleansing that apply for all types of skin at any age: NEVER USE SOAP and BE GENTLE.

Choosing a cleanser depends on your type of skin and your preference for a specific product as determined by its feel, its aroma, and its effectiveness. Cleansers come in four basic forms: creams, milks, gels, and foaming cleansers. Creams are heavy and thick and contain more oil than water. Milky cleansers are a balanced formulation of oil and water and are thinner than a cream. Gels are usually oil free and have a thickened, gel-like consistency. Foaming cleansers contain ingredients that create suds. There are some foaming cleansers available now that do not contain detergent or soap and offer an alternative for those people who like their cleanser to have a foaming action.

Soap and detergents are not an option as facial cleansers because they are very alkaline, they destroy the protective acid pH mantle of the skin, and they strip the skin of its natural, protective oils. The regular use of soap or detergent contributes to the premature ageing of the skin because of the soap or detergent's drying effects. Dr. Peter Pugliese, dermatologist and author of <u>Advanced Professional Skin Care</u>, states, "Using soap as the major facial cleansing agent has serious drawbacks. To what extent it adds to wrinkle formation has not been determined exactly, but there is no doubt that it is a contributing agent." Be certain to read the labels of cleansers, and avoid those that contain soap or detergent. (Hint: if your cleanser is leaving your face 'squeaky clean,' it is too strong).

TONERS

The toner is used after cleansing. Toners were originally designed to wipe the face clean of any trace of the cleanser. These old formulas usually contained alcohol. This not only removed every bit of cleanser but also every bit of natural skin oil, which made the toners drying and sometimes irritating to the skin. Times have changed, and the better toners are now formulated without alcohol. My favorite toners are ones that are simply formulated and contain aloe and/or herbal extracts.

A good toner will remove any residue left by the cleanser, reestablish the pH balance of the skin (if it has been disrupted by the cleanser), condition and 'tone' the skin, and prepare the skin for moisturizing. To use a toner, saturate a cotton ball and then gently wipe the face and neck. Using a cotton ball is more effective that just patting the toner on the face because the cotton ball will lift off and take away any residue or remaining soil.

MOISTURIZERS

Moisturizing is the third step of a basic skin care routine. Moisturizers are most effective when applied after the skin has been hydrated by water from a shower, a bath, facial compresses, or facial misting. The purpose of moisturizing is to form a protective barrier that prevents moisture loss and to guard against the effects of harsh weather and environmental conditions that can damage the skin, such as pollutants. (A well-formulated moisturizer will do this without clogging the pores.) If the moisturizer contains a good humectant (such as glycerin or hyaluronic acid), it will hold moisture next to the skin, which is very beneficial to counteracting dryness and the signs of ageing. Moisturizers can make the skin feel softer and smoother while nurturing it with active ingredients such as vitamins, herbal extracts, and essential oils.

Moisturizers tend to be the most elaborate of the three basic products and are usually the most expensive. They are formulated using an emulsion (combination) of water and oil for a smooth, creamy consistency (with the exception of the new 'oil-free' moisturizers) and serve to imitate our own natural skin protective system – the sweat and oil glands that excrete both water and oil on the surface of the skin. The 'richer' moisturizers have more oil. The 'lighter' ones have more water. There are moisturizers formulated as night creams and others as day creams. Generally, the difference is the night cream is 'richer' and contains more active, nourishing ingredients, and the day cream is lighter and designed to be more protective. Not all manufacturers make both a day and a night cream, and there is a difference of opinion about the use and need of these types of creams. Some feel that a day and a night cream are not necessary and that one cream with do fine for both situations. Others feel it is important to sleep with the face clean so that it can breathe and rejuvenate. Still others feel this is the time to nurture the skin with special ingredients. This may ultimately be a matter of personal choice. However, if you choose to use a night cream, use it sparingly. A thick coat prevents the skin from respirating and excreting properly while you are sleeping.

There are two rules of thumb for using a moisturizer. First, use it only when and where you need it. If you have an oily forehead, don't put any moisturizer there. This also holds true for the nose and chin. Use your discretion. If your skin feels tight and dry, you need to use a moisturizer. If you have very oily skin, you may not need one at all. Secondly, the type of moisturizer you are using may need to be changed with the seasons or with a change of environment. If you are in extreme cold with winds, you need a 'richer,' heavier moisturizer for more protection. If it is summertime and you are in humid weather, you may need a moisturizer only on your cheeks. There is flexibility with using a moisturizer, depending on your skin type and the situation. The important thing to know is that you do not <u>always</u> have to wear a moisturizer <u>all</u> over your face <u>all</u> of the time.

SKIN CARE PROGRAM GUIDELINES

FOR ALL SKIN TYPES

*A*ll skin types will benefit from a pre-cleansing technique that is called 'facial compressing,' and it should be the first step in any cleansing process. This technique was described by a friend of mine as serving the same purpose as soaking the dishes before washing them. In essence, facial compressing begins to soften and loosen that which will be cleansed away – making the cleansing process easier and more effective.

The technique is simple and takes only a moment. Fill the basin with warm water and lean over it while you use a clean washcloth to hold the water to your face. Apply at least ten compresses. While your face is still damp, apply your cleanser and proceed with the cleansing process.

Facial compressing can be made a little more elaborate and a lot more enjoyable with three to five drops of lavender essential oil. Not only is the lavender excellent for the skin, it also has a beautiful fragrance which relaxes and calms the psyche.

NORMAL SKIN

The goal of a skin care program for the lucky person with normal skin is to maintain this well-balanced condition with proper care. Normal skin has more freedom than the other skin types to experiment with different types of cleansers, be they oil free, milky, or a soap-free foaming cleanser. Oil free cleansers are more appropriate for younger, normal skin (teen to twenty-five years), and the milky cleansers are good for maturing, normal skin. Normal skin should be cleansed and toned twice a day, in the morning and before going to sleep. Use a light moisturizer only where needed.

OILY SKIN

People with oily skin need to resist the temptation to over-cleanse their skin by using either too harsh a cleanser, cleansing too often, or cleansing too vigorously. This not only damages the skin, it also aggravates and stimulates the oily condition. Oily skin needs to be gently cleansed twice a day – in the morning and before going to bed. Using cool compresses in the pre-cleanse step will help to sedate the oil glands. Younger oily skin should avoid any cleansers that contain oil. Best suited for this type of skin are the cleansing gels. For maturing oily skin, a milky cleanser can be used to its advantage, as long as the cleanser is well formualted and will rinse well from the skin. Oily skin at any age should avoid heavy cream cleansers. Follow the cleansing with an aloe or herbal extract based toner.

Younger oily skin may not need a moisturizer at all. However, if one is used, it must be oil free. Mature oily skin may be dehydrated (lacking water) and will benefit from the protection and hydrating qualities of a moisturizer. The moisturizer can be oil free or a light cream and should be used sparingly only in the areas that need it.

DRY SKIN

Dry skin requires a program that will protect it from moisture loss and harsh conditions such as wind, extreme temperatures, or the sun. It needs to be well hydrated both internally and externally. Dry skin, whether lacking oil, lacking water, or both, will greatly benefit from ample, warm facial compresses because they stimulate glandular function (water and oil) and hydrate the skin. I recommend cleansing one time a day for dry skin. Time after time, I have seen dry-skinned people benefit from only a single cleansing – at night. In the morning, splash the face with warm water or use facial compresses again. Pat dry excess moisture and then apply a moisturizer. Milky cleansers are the best for dry skin although creamy cleansers are also appropriate. Never, never use soap on dry skin. Be certain the toner that you are using is formulated for dry skin.

Dry skin needs a medium, well-balanced moisturizer with a very good humectant for regular use. However, if dry skin is exposed to cold or wind or high heats, a heavier moisturizer should be used.

COMBINATION SKIN

Combination skin is the most common skin type and needs a program to help balance the two types of skin. Almost everyone has a slightly more oily 'T zone' (forehead, nose, and sometimes, chin). The cheeks and the area around the eyes are usually drier. Cleanse twice a day – morning and evening. Use warm, but not hot, facial compresses. Depending on the degree of difference between these two zones, you may be able to use the same cleanser for the whole face or you may have to use two separate cleansers. If you are trying to use only one cleanser, use the one for the least oily area – dry or normal. It is better for your complexion to under-cleanse the oily part than to over-cleanse the drier part. Most cases of combination skin are not extreme, and I have had clients do very well using products designed for 'normal skin' that seemed to help balance the two zones. The toner requires the same guidelines; depending on the degree of difference in the two areas of skin, you may need to use two different formulas. A moisturizer should be used on the dry or normal areas, and the oily areas may not require any moisturizer at all.

SENSITIVE SKIN

Sensitive skin must be handled gently and individually. Sensitivities can vary. A simple, gentle skin care program seems to work the best. It may be necessary to try several different product lines to find one that works effectively without irritating. Avoid artificial colors and fragrances – they are known irritants.

Sensitive skin fares better when cleansed only one time a day – in the evening (see Dry Skin). In the pre-cleanse step, use warm (not hot) facial compresses. For cleansing, use a gentle milky cleanser. Avoid cleansers with complicated ingredients. Use a toner lightly. It may be necessary to dilute the toner to make it gentler. Pay attention. If your skin becomes upset at any phase of your skin care program – the cleanser, the temperature of the water, the number of times you cleanse, the toner, or the moisturizer – you will need to change the program.

Sensitive skin requires good protection because it can be easily upset and damaged by extreme heat or cold, pollution, and other environmental conditions. Just like other products for sensitive skin, the moisturizer should be simply formulated. Some active ingredients may be too active for very sensitive skin. It is also wise to switch moisturizers periodically, because sensitive skin has a tendency to develop allergic reactions easier and sooner than other skin types, and the skin can become sensitized from using the same product for long periods of time.

ACNEIC SKIN

Acneic skin or skin with blemishes needs very gentle care. After all, it is quite upset. Use cool to slightly warm facial compresses before cleansing. This skin type should be cleansed well, two times a day, morning and evening. Do not use a cream cleanser on acne skin and DO NOT OVER CLEANSE with a strong, drying cleanser. Cleansing gels and some well-formulated cleansing milks can be used. Use a toner specially made for this skin type. Aloe and herbal extract based toners are excellent. Look for additional ingredients that can calm and purify the skin. Moisturizers may not be necessary unless the skin is dehydrated. In this case, an oil free moisturizer should be used.

AGEING SKIN

Ageing skin should be treated gently and nurtured. Though all of us will develop ageing skin as the years go by, if properly cared for, our skin can have a vibrant appearance and look beautiful at every age.

Ageing skin is losing its moisture content and its glandular function is slowing down, so plenty of warm compresses are in order. Do a thorough cleansing only one time a day using either a milky or creamy cleanser and follow with a toner designed for dry or mature skin. Use the 'rinse and splash method' in the morning as described for dry skin.

Ageing skin needs all the benefits a good moisturizer can provide – effective active ingredients such as essential oils, a good humectant for hydration, and anti-oxidant vitamins and herbs to fight free radical damage.

SPECIAL CONSIDERATIONS FOR MATURING SKIN

(AGEING PREVENTION)

*T*hrough the course of our lives, our skin will change. It will pass from the soft and delicate characteristics of baby skin to childhood's smooth, velvety texture and resilient nature. It will go through the teenage years known for the problems and through the twenties when our skin begins to mature. By our thirties, we may notice it becoming drier with the first signs of wrinkles, and by forty-something...our skin is ageing.

As the skin ages, it characteristically becomes drier and loses its elasticity. The skin's rejuvenating capacity (cell renewal) slows down, and the oxygen and nutrient supply decreases with a reduction in circulation. Protective oil (sebum) production decreases. These changes take place in the dermal layer of the skin. How fast and to what extent this dermal layer changes depends on three things: your age, your heredity, and your lifestyle.

On the surface of the skin, as the cells work their way from the dermal layer, they are thicker and more dense and have decreased ability to retain moisture. The cells are not well lubricated, because of the decrease of oil. This gives mature skin its drier appearance.

All of the items listed in "A Checklist for Beautiful Skin" are crucial considerations for ageing skin. In fact, if an effective program is put into practice early in life and <u>before</u> the skin begins to show signs of ageing, many of the symptoms of ageing skin could be avoided for a long time.

In addition to the checklist, there are other considerations for mature skin:

- **Avoid over-manipulation.** Over-manipulation refers to heavy scrubbing, heavy facial massage, and over-stretching the skin while applying make-up or skin care products. The facial skin does not have much ability to 'bounce back,' particularly as we get older. This over-manipulation encourages the skin to wrinkle and sag.

- **Avoid over-cleansing.** Over-cleansing can mean two things: washing the face more times than is necessary for the particular skin type and/or using too harsh a cleanser. Over-cleansing is destructive to the health and function of the skin because it strips away the natural oils and disrupts the protective mantle. This can lead to both dryness and irritation, which is particularly damaging to ageing skin.

- **Beware of extreme weight loss.** Dieting can affect the skin in two ways. First, most dieting programs are low in fats and oils. The skin needs oils to stay soft and supple. Secondly, as we get older and our skin's elasticity decreases, it is not able to accommodate extreme swings in weight. A great loss of weight can leave heavily wrinkled and saggy skin. If you are dieting, try to lose the weight slowly, and if you must exclude fats and oils, supplement your diet with a product rich in essential fatty acids.

- **Give special care to the eye area.** The delicate skin around the eyes is the first to show signs of ageing. Here, the skin has few of the oil and sweat glands necessary to keep it conditioned. It is also constantly moving, very thin skinned, and very sensitive to mistreatment. Preventative care and proper skin care habits can delay the visible signs of ageing around the eyes. In addition to the other considerations mentioned, it is recommended that whenever you are applying moisturizers in the eye area, pat or press them in place to avoid stretching the tissue. When you are in the sun, wear sunglasses large enough to cover the entire eye area. The lenses must be the type that block ultra violet rays. In cold weather and the wind, use a heavier moisturizer for protection. Try not to rub your eyes. It stretches the skin and encourages the orbital fat to herniate and form bags. Lastly, avoid using 'kleenex' type tissues around the eyes. They are made of wood bits that can irritate the skin.

- **Provide nutritional supplementation.** To combat the dryness and damage associated with ageing skin, the diet must include plenty of fluids (water, juices, herbal teas), oils (essential fatty acids), and anti-oxidants. Anti-oxidants inhibit free radical damage that has been caused by exposure to sun, smog, and cigarette smoke as well as by the body's normal chemical processes. Some anti-oxidant nutrients are vitamins A, C, and E, selenium, bioflavinoids, beta carotene, and pycnogenol.

SPECIAL TREATMENTS

$\mathcal{I}$n addition to the basic skin care routine of cleansing, toning, and moisturizing, there are special treatments that you can do to benefit your skin. Nature offers a variety of safe, healthy, and effective means of nurturing and encouraging skin vitality for skin of all types. Steaming treatments, exfoliants, aromatherapy treatments, masks, eye creams, and facial misting can be incorporated into a daily, weekly, or monthly program.

STEAMING

Steaming is used in a skin care routine because it super-hydrates the skin, softens dead skin cells, relaxes the facial muscles, and 'opens' the pores for deep and thorough cleansing. It also increases circulation to the skin and encourages cell metabolism.

Small, facial steaming machines are available for home use from drug and department stores. I recommend them instead of the face-over-the-pot-of-water method. In the latter, the steam doesn't last long enough to be of much use, and the face can easily be burned by the first burst of steam. The small facial steamers are much better – safer and more effective.

While every skin type can benefit from steaming, be sure to follow these guidelines. Normal, oily, and combination skin (if the dry part is not too dry) can be steamed once a week for about ten minutes. Acne skin can steam more often if it has been determined that it is beneficial. Sensitive, ageing, and dry skin can be steamed once a week or every other week for two to five minutes – being certain that the steam is not too hot on the face. Although steaming is beneficial for these skin types, steaming too often may not be. Every skin type should protect the delicate area around the eyes and the lips with a moisturizer during the steaming process. If you have a couperose condition (distended capillaries) on your face, this area should also be protected with a moisturizer.

EXFOLIANTS

The concept of exfoliants and their role in skin care has been around quite a while. Their purpose is to encourage the removal of dead skin cells and debris from the surface of the skin, revealing a softer, smoother complexion. In the past, the most common exfoliants were the ones with a grainy texture, often called 'scrubs.' I never liked scrubs for the facial skin because many of them were poorly formulated and were so rough that they damaged the skin. In addition, the consumer was not well-educated in the use of the exfoliants, causing more skin damage than improvement.

Today, however, there are two new types of exfoliants available and they are a boon to natural skin care. Green papaya and alpha hydroxy acids offer treatments that are gentle, and very effective – far more effective than the granular exfoliants. The green papaya digests 'dead' protein (dead skin cells) with an enzyme called *papain*. This results in softer, smoother skin. Alpha hydroxy acids dissolve a protein, glue-like substance that holds dead skin cells together on the surface of the skin. Regular and consistent use of alpha hydroxy acids result in the exfoliation of these skin cells, revealing smoother, softer skin, improved texture, and a reduction in fine lines and wrinkles.

Each type of skin can benefit from these new exfoliants, especially sun-damaged and ageing skin. Both of these exfoliants are being formulated in masks, liquid treatments, moisturizers, and lotions. Sensitive-skinned people may not be able to use them because the ingredients are too 'active,' but it is worth a try. Those with acneic skin may notice an improvement in their condition.

AROMATHERAPY TREATMENTS

Aromatherapy (essential oils) have been used throughout history by people all over the world to enhance their health and beauty. Essential oils are extracted from plant material – the petals, roots, leaves, barks, stalks, or seeds.

The term 'aromatherapy' was first used in the 1920's by a French chemist named R.M. Gattefosse. It literally means 'fragrant remedy.' Today, aromatherapy is defined as a treatment using the essential oils from aromatic plants for the purpose of restoring or enhancing health and beauty. Its influence is being felt in the fields of medicine, psychology, and cosmetology.

Cosmetically, essential oils are a delight to use because of their enticing fragrances and their profound effect in skin care. Aromatherapy is a marvelous way to pamper the skin, and virtually all types of skin can benefit from it. The effectiveness of essential oils is due to their ability to penetrate the skin. They have a very small and simple molecular structure, and when applied to the skin, they pass into the fluid surrounding the cells beneath the skin's surface.

There are commercial aromatherapy facial oils available for every skin type. These treatments are an appropriate blend of the concentrated essentials oils diluted in a base oil. Undiluted essential oils should not be used on the face, because they may cause irritation. I recommend using aromatherapy facial oils as a night treatment, to be applied after the face has been cleansed. Only a few drops are needed. Place the oil in the palm of your hand, rub your hands together, and then press and pat your face and neck. Certain essential oils have rejuvenating properties, others are calming or balancing. The best essential oils used in aromatherapy for cosmetic purposes are from flowers such as lavender, geranium, chamomile, and rose.

Aromatherapy treatments seem to appeal to everyone. They are very special and effective. Not only are they wonderful for the skin, they are also wonderful for the psyche. The most popular cosmetic essential oils include:

- **Lavender.** Lavender is considered to be the most useful and versatile of all the essential oils. It is soothing, antiseptic, anti-inflammatory, and has balancing qualities that make it invaluable for skin care. Lavender is one of the few oils that can be applied undiluted (neat) to the skin, and few people are allergic to it. It is excellent for the treatment of acne because it inhibits bacteria, soothes the skin, helps to balance the over-active sebaceous glands, and helps to reduce scarring by stimulating the growth of healthy new cells. It is beneficial for all types of skin, including ageing skin. It is soothing to the psyche and relaxes the nervous system.

- **Chamomile.** Chamomile's qualities are soothing, calming, and anti-inflammatory. It is an analgesic and a disinfectant and it is very gentle in nature. Chamomile is especially good for dry, sensitive skin, and because it has the ability to shrink small blood vessels, it can help reduce the redness due to enlarged capillaries. Chamomile is an anti-depressant and relieves irritability and insomnia. It calms the nerves.

- **Geranium.** Geranium is astringent, antiseptic, and it promotes speedy healing. It is excellent in balancing the production of sebum, so it is well-suited for all skin types, especially combination skin. Geranium has an antidepressant, uplifting, and calming effect on the psyche.

- **Rose.** Rose is considered the 'queen' of essential oils. It is good for all types of skin but especially for dry, sensitive, or ageing skin. It is an excellent antiseptic and can help diminish enlarged capillaries when used regularly. It is a gentle yet powerful anti-depressant. It soothes the nerves and is renowned for its aphrodisiac qualities. It is one of the most expensive oils.

- **Sandalwood.** Sandalwood is good for all types of skin. It is excellent for dry, dehydrated skin and beneficial for oily and acne skin as well. It is soothing, inhibits bacterial growth, and is slightly astringent. Sandalwood is warming and relaxing and is an aphrodisiac.

- **Ylang Ylang.** Ylang Ylang is suitable for both oily and dry skin because it has a balancing effect on the secretion of sebum. It is soothing. It affects the psyche by counteracting anger and frustration. It is considered an aphrodisiac and a euphoric.

- **Frankincense.** Frankincense is an excellent oil for mature skin because of its rejuvenating properties. It is distilled from the resin of the Boswellia tree in Arabia. It is calming to the emotions.

- **Jasmine.** Jasmine can be used for all types of skin. It has a toning, antiseptic quality. It is soothing and excellent for dry, sensitive skin. Jasmine relaxes the mind and helps to alleviate anger, nervousness, and worries.

- **Neroli (Orange Blossom).** Neroli is known for its rejuvenating qualities and is especially good for dry and mature skin. It calms the psyche and has aphrodisiac qualities. It is a very expensive oil, and its aroma has been described as "hauntingly beautiful."

MASKS

A facial mask is a special treatment that is available for all skin types to enjoy. Masks are formulated in a variety of ways, depending on the manufacturer's design, and serve the purpose of moisturizing, tightening, cleansing, soothing, stimulating, or nourishing the skin.

Clay-based masks are considered tightening and cleansing masks because of the clay's ability to absorb oil and toxins. Some clays are very high in minerals which will nourish the skin. Clay masks are often formulated with a variety of special ingredients. They can be used by people with normal skin (once a month) or with oily or problem skin (once a week).

Those with problem skin may benefit from using clay masks more often. The clay paste should be applied thickly to the skin for about fifteen minutes. A clay mask should not be allowed to dry completely because it will begin to draw moisture out of the skin. If the mask starts to dry before fifteen minutes, mist it to keep it damp.

Cream masks are designed to soothe, moisturize, and nourish the skin. They do not contain clay. They are especially good for dry, ageing, or sensitive skin and depending on the formulation are to be used about once a week. Normal skin will also benefit from cream masks, particularly when it feels drier than usual as a result of environmental exposure or a season change.

EYE CREAMS

Eye creams are designed to protect and nurture the delicate skin around the eyes. Because this area has few oil glands and because the eyes are constantly moving, this is usually the first place that the signs of age begin to show. Eye creams are meant to prevent this from happening prematurely. They are available in formulations ranging from lightweight oils to heavy creams. Eye gels are also available. Personal preference should be your guide.

People of all skin types should begin using an eye treatment around the age of twenty-five or sooner if necessary. Even people with oily or problem skin can use this treatment, although they should use the lighter formulas. Eye creams, oils, and gels should be applied sparingly around the eye in a pat-and-press method. Do not rub or stretch the skin. If you use too

much product or get the product in the eye, it can cause puffi-
ness. Eye treatments can be worn during the day and at night
while you sleep. The lighter weight treatments are better during
the day so as not to disrupt eye make-up. The heavier ones are
excellent at night after you have hydrated your skin with facial
compresses and the cleansing process.

FACIAL MISTING

Facial misting is a delightful and refreshing skin care
habit. Facial misters are small bottles with a pump sprayer. The
contents can be just plain water or a special blend of water
with herbal extracts, water with essential oils, floral waters
(hydrosols), or aloe vera. The primary function of facial misters
is to hydrate the skin. I have had many clients whose facial dryness, including fine lines, almost disappeared with regular
facial misting. However, in order for it to be effective, it must
be used in conjunction with a good moisturizer that contains a
good humectant. The spray that the misters emit is very fine and
will not disturb make-up. Facial misting is good for all skin
types, especially dry and ageing, and can be used as often as
desired, at least three times a day – morning, noon, and night.

SKIN CARE
FOR THE BODY

*W*hen discussing skin care, we generally think of the facial skin. However, skin care should not stop at the neck – the body skin also needs care and attention and will benefit from a program of external cleansing, stimulating, conditioning/nourishing, protecting, and exfoliating.

CLEANSING

We cleanse our bodies to remove the excreted wastes from the surface of the skin and to remove accumulated dust and dirt. This can be accomplished with a gentle scrubbing and rinsing with water.

Americans over-clean their skin with their exaggerated and frequent use of soap. This is not a practice that is followed worldwide. Soap is very harsh and causes the skin to become irritated and superficially dry. It destroys the acid pH mantle on the surface of the skin and removes the natural oils, both of which were designed to provide protection. It takes time for the acid mantle and oil to re-establish themselves, once removed, and if they are daily washed away, the protection cannot be at its optimum level.

Most of us do not lead the kind of life that necessitates daily bathing, yet often this is our practice. I strongly advise against daily soaping of the entire body or soaking in a tub of soapy water. Certain areas which have become soiled or that perspire heavily might be washed daily, but avoid washing the other areas that do not need it. The shins, for instance, do not have many oil glands, and they will become very dry if soap is used regularly on them. If this concept of not soaping the skin seems foreign and unappealing to you, give it a try for one week. For your daily bath or shower, simply rinse the skin with water. Rinsing is also cleansing, but it is not stripping. In the time of one week, your skin will feel softer and it will be in a healthier condition.

For the areas that may require a little soap, choose a gentle liquid. If you have particularly sensitive or dry skin, dilute it to one part soap to six parts water. Keep it in a squeeze bottle for easy application and use it sparingly. Rinse off all soap very, very well. Remember, soap is very drying to the skin and contributes to visible ageing.

The shower and the bath, America's most common ways to cleanse the body, are hydrotherapy treatments – providing the benefits of water and the temperature you choose. Warm water has a sedating and relaxing effect, and cool water is stimulating and invigorating. Showers are quick and easy and are the most popular. The bath, famous throughout history for its therapeutic and social functions, can be a luxurious and relaxing activity. The temperature of a long bath should always be moderate – if it is too hot it will encourage capillary distension, causing veins to appear red and 'spidery' on the surface of the skin. It can also drain your energy and dry your skin. If the temperature is too cold, it can depress the body's circulation. (Hot and cold baths can be used therapeutically but only if used for short periods of time.)

STIMULATING

Stimulating the skin supports the skin's many functions and can even increase their capabilities. This stimulation can be accomplished by dry brush massage, manual massage, brisk drying with a rough terry towel, or use of a washcloth with a grain meal scrub (not soap). Scrubs are exfoliating agents that can be used for the body if they are gentle and the 'texture' in them is derived from nut meals, grain meals, jojoba beads, coarse salt, or something with similar soft edges. (Do not use any product that uses sharp-edged substances such as walnut or almond shells.)

The best method to stimulate the skin is dry brush massage. Dry brush massage has been used in one form or another for ages by cultures all over the world. It is superb for the skin as well as for general health. Dry brush massage cleanses the skin without removing the protective pH mantle or natural skin oils. It stimulates the hormone and oil-producing glands in the dermal layer. By sloughing off the top layer of dead skin cells, it opens the pores and assists the respirating function. It can assist in the breaking up of fat deposits. Circulation is stimulated, bringing more vital nutrients and oxygen to nourish the skin as well as underlying organs and tissues. Rough skin, especially on the upper arms, can be smoothed and softened by dry brush massage.

The skin is our largest eliminative organ, excreting one-third of the body's toxins. It works in conjunction with the other cleansing organs such as the kidneys, the alimentary canal, the liver, the lungs, and the mucous membranes. The less active the skin, the greater is the work load put on the other organs. Dry brush massage benefits our general health by stimulating the lymphatic system and increasing the skin's ability as an eliminative organ, aiding the entire body.

Dry brush massage is best done before a bath or shower so the dead skin cells will be rinsed off the body. It is done with a long-handled, natural vegetable bristle brush that should be used exclusively for this purpose. These brushes are available at natural food stores. Begin brushing the extremities and work in circular motions toward the heart. Brush all of your skin, except the face. Periodically, wash the brush and let it dry thoroughly before using it again. Do not brush irritated skin and be gentle with dry or sensitive skin. This very simple yet invaluable skin care exercise will leave you feeling warm and revitalized. It is recommended to be practiced daily and will produce remarkable results.

CONDITIONING/NOURISHING

The skin is best nourished from the food we eat, the water we drink, and the air we breathe. However, external treatments can condition and nourish the skin as well. Because the skin is capable of absorbing substances that are of a small enough molecular structure, there is value to well-formulated, nutritive body lotions, body oils, herbal wraps, and body masks. Just as these types of products are so carefully selected for the face, so also should they be carefully selected for the body – the principles of the considerations are the same.

PROTECTING

Protection from the conditions of the environment is necessary to prevent skin irritation, damage, and moisture loss. The sun's damaging effects can cause burning, blistering, premature wrinkling, and skin cancer. Your skin can be protected from the sun by staying out of the sun, wearing sunblock, and wearing protective clothing such as long sleeves, long pants, hats, and sunglasses. Excessive wind, salt water and air, extremes in weather, and pollution can be drying and damaging, particularly for sensitive skin. The skin can be somewhat protected in these conditions with a good body lotion or oil and clothing, but it is best to try to avoid over-exposure to these situations.

Daily use of a body lotion or oil will help to keep the skin soft and supple and protect against moisture loss. It is best applied after a shower or bath. At this time, the skin has been hydrated and the oil in the lotion or body oil will seal in the moisture. Pat dry, leaving a slight amount of moisture, and apply a thin film to the body, especially on the parts that are exposed to the elements.

EXFOLIATING

Exfoliation is the assistance to the sloughing off process of dead skin cells on the surface of the skin. Our skin does this naturally but as we grow older there is more dead skin cell buildup and the sloughing off process slows down. Exfoliating simply aids this natural process. Dry brush massage is an excellent and effective method of exfoliation. Other mechanical methods are loofahs, scrubs, or pumice stones (for calloused areas only).

Very gentle methods of exfoliation can be used on the body with products that contain either green papaya or alpha hydroxy acids. These are described in more detail in "Special Treatments" under "Exfoliants." Both green papaya and alpha hydroxy acids will leave the skin feeling silky, soft, and smooth. They are excellent for sun-damaged or ageing skin.

SPECIAL CARE FOR THE HANDS

*B*ecause the hands are constantly exposed to the elements, as is the face, they begin to show wear and tear and ageing sooner than other parts of the body. There are a few things that you can do to help keep your hands soft and attractive.

- Protect your hands from strong detergents, cleaning products, and frequent immersion in water by wearing rubber gloves. These conditions remove protective oils and can cause dryness and irritation and possible allergic reaction.

- Use a hand cream or lotion every time you wash your hands and massage it into the cuticles. This will help prevent dryness and cracking.

- To prevent 'age' spots on the backs of your hands, keep them out of the sun and protect them with a sunblock of SPF 15.

- Beware of allergic reactions to nail cosmetics, especially polishes. The most common reaction is a rash or itching around the nail. Some people have experienced the nail plate separating from the nail bed. Avoid nail polishes that contain formaldehyde – it is a common allergen.

- Do not use nail polish remover more than once a week. Using it frequently will cause drying of the nail and the surrounding tissue.

- Avoid traumatic blows to the nail plate as well as the

base of the nail. It can cause permanent damage and result in a deformed nail.

- After a bath or shower is an excellent time to groom your nails. Clean under the free edge, gently push back the cuticle while the skin is soft from bathing, and clip off any loose skin or hangnails.

SUPER NATURAL INGREDIENTS FOR SKIN CARE

In the world of natural cosmetic ingredients, there are a few that stand out above the rest for their effectiveness and desirability in skin care products. When you are shopping, read the labels and look for the following exceptional ingredients. They will be found in cleansers, toners, moisturizers, and special treatments. (Also be armed with a cosmetic ingredient book such as Ruth Winter's A Consumer's Dictionary of Cosmetic Ingredients – so you will know about the other ingredients included in a product.)

ALOE VERA is a tropical plant whose sharp-edged, triangular leaves contain a viscous, transparent gel that promotes healing and aids in the stimulation of cellular renewal. The gel contains amino acids, minerals, vitamins, carbohydrates, and enzymes. It is soothing, moisturizing, and toning for all types of skin. It also has antibiotic, anti-bacterial, and anti-inflammatory qualities.

ALPHA HYDROXY ACIDS (AHA's) are a group of non-toxic fruit acids. Glycolic acid is currently the most widely used. However, the others in the group, such as lactic, tartaric, citric, and malic acids, are finding their way into use as well. Alpha hydroxy acids dissolve and loosen the protein glue-like substance that binds together the corneocytes (dead skin cells) on the surface of the skin. As these dead skin cells are removed, a smoother and younger-appearing complexion is revealed. The regular and consistent use of alpha hydroxy acids has been shown to soften fine lines and wrinkles, improve dry skin, help control blemishes, and reduce discoloration.

CLAY is rich in mineral content and is excellent for the skin when used in masks. It has an ability to absorb toxins and cleanse. It increases circulation and revitalizes the skin.

ESSENTIAL OILS are discussed in "Special Treatments" under 'Aromatherapy Treatments.'

GLYCERINE is a natural humectant that can come from either animal or vegetable sources. It is effective for holding water next to the skin to help keep it from becoming dry. It also aids in the spreadability of a product. Glycerin, formulated in high percentages, may attract moisture from the skin (which could lead to dryness), so cosmetic products should only contain less than twenty per cent.

GREEN PAPAYA is rich in a proteolytic (digesting) enzyme that when used on the skin encourages the sloughing off of old, dead skin cells. (Interestingly, the enzyme only 'digests' the damaged or dead skin cells.) This reveals a new, softer skin. Green papaya has been shown to be effective in neutralizing free radicals.

HERBAL EXTRACTS have been used in cosmetics for thousands of years for their softening, soothing, protecting, stimulating, and rejuvenating properties. Herbal extracts are made by extracting the properties of the herb with a solvent, usually water or alcohol, although glycerin and vinegar are also used. The herbs that are used in cosmetics are too numerous to list here; however, listed are some of the most popular:

> **Arnica.** Soothes skin irritation; purifies and promotes healing.

> **Calendula.** Cleansing, soothing and healing; anti-inflammatory; stimulates circulation.

> **Chamomile.** Anti-inflammatory, soothing; accelerates healing; softening; regenerative; antioxidant.

> **Comfrey.** Soothing and healing because of its allantoin and carotene contents; moisturizing, anti-inflammatory; promotes cell regeneration; astringent and cleansing.

> **Elderflower.** Reduces inflammation; slightly astringent, cleansing.

> **Ginkgo Biloba.** Rich in a flavonoid complex; anti-inflammatory qualities; increases circulation and cellular activity; powerful anti-oxidant.

> **Ginseng.** May stimulate the formation of new cells; tones, rejuvenates, balances; anti-oxidant abilities.

Horsetail. Rich in silica, a mineral that is necessary for healthy skin and hair; astringent properties; tones.

Lavender. Balances; cell regenerator; promotes rapid healing.

Nettle. Purifies and tones; rich in minerals; stimulates circulation.

Peppermint. Purifies; has astringent qualities.

Rosemary. Stimulates circulation, rejuvenates, tones; antiseptic.

St. Johnswort. Used to tone, strengthen, and heal; has a calming quality.

Witch Hazel. Astringent; reduces inflammation.

Yarrow. Slightly astringent; tones.

HYALURONIC ACID is a polysaccharide (complex carbohydrate) that is a gel-like, natural component of human skin in the dermal layer. Collagen and elastin are surrounded by hyaluronic acid, and its water-binding quality helps maintain moisture and flexibility. It can hold 500-plus times its own weight in water, making it an exceptional humectant and moisturizer.

PLANT OILS were, historically, the first cosmetic ingredients known to be in constant demand. They were used extensively to make soap, cold creams, and lotions. Although there was a period of time when their use in cosmetics diminished, today they are back in favor, offering emollient, nurturing, soothing, and moisturizing benefits to the skin without clogging the pores. The following are popular plant oils for cosmetic use:

Avocado Oil. Excellent emollient with some sunscreen properties; easily absorbed into the skin; contains vitamins A, D, and E; helps to smooth and soften; excellent for mature skin.

Almond Oil. A soothing emollient and skin softener; excellent for mature skin.

Macadamia Nut Oil. Excellent for dry and mature skin because of its palmitoleic acid – a substance found in the sebum of young people. As we age, the amount of palmitoleic acid decreases in the skin.

Squalene Oil. From the olive tree; extremely compatible with the skin; good for all skin types, especially for dry and sensitive.

Jojoba Oil Comes from the bean of a desert bush; excellent for the skin; soothes, moisturizes, and nurtures; has the unique quality of being a liquid wax, which helps prevent rancidity. It is said to very closely resemble the natural oil of our skin, sebum. Because of this compatibility, it can break up the sebum in clogged pores. It is non-greasy and it nourishes, lubricates, and softens the skin..

Olive Oil. Rich in vitamins; nourishing and calming.

Wheat Germ Oil. Rich in vitamin E, pro-vitamin A and vitamin F; nutritive, moisturizing; easily penetrates the skin; regenerating and nourishing.

Sesame Oil. Rich in vitamins.

Soybean Oil. Rich in vitamins, lecithin; easily absorbed into the skin; nourishes, softens, and moisturizes.

PYCNOGENOL is a flavonoid from the bark of the maritime pine tree. It is also found in beans, grapes, cranberries, and other fruits and vegetables, but not in as concentrated a form as in the pine tree. It is a powerful anti-oxidant, being more active than both vitamin E and vitamin C. It strengthens capillary walls and binds to collagen to help prevent wrinkles and damage to the skin.

SEAWEED (algae) is rich in vitamins and minerals that are beneficial and rejuvenating to the skin. It also has free radical scavenging and detoxifying capabilities.

SHEA BUTTER is also called karite butter. It is an exceptionally rich vegetable fat with excellent moisturizing and lubricating qualities.

VITAMINS are defined as "any of a group of organic (carbon containing) substances essential in small quantities to promote one or more specific and essential biochemical reactions within the living cell for normal metabolism and health." The vitamins that are used in cosmetics are used primarily for their anti-oxidant, free radical scavenging capabilities and their rejuvenating properties. Listed here are the most popular:

Vitamin E's most valuable contribution is its ability to slow down the ageing and degeneration of skin cells. It promotes cellular renewal, skin elasticity, and healing. Its excellent antioxidant qualities fight free radicals and keep products fresh for longer periods of time.

Vitamin F is excellent for hydration and lubrication of skin cells, keeping the skin soft, smooth, and youthful.

Vitamin A is necessary for tissue generation, repair, and maintenance. It accelerates the formation of new cells, prevents increased keratinization (thickening) of the skin, deters excessive dryness, and regulates glandular functions in the skin. It also has anti-oxidant properties.

Vitamin C is an excellent anti-oxidant that protects skin cells. It fights infections and supports collagen production.

WATER is one of the most important ingredients in a cosmetic formula for the skin because moisture is the key to keeping skin youthful and healthy. Vital in keeping the skin soft and supple, water is used in creams and lotions as part of an emulsion (water and oil combined). Water also helps carry active ingredients into the skin.

GLOSSARY OF TERMS

ANTISEPTICS inhibit the growth of germs and microorganisms.

ASTRINGENTS have a tightening, constricting action on the skin.

ANTI-OXIDANTS are substances that inhibit oxidation. The term anti-oxidant is frequently linked with the term 'free radicals' these days because anti-oxidants protect living cells from free radical damage. Anti-oxidants such as vitamin A (including beta carotene), vitamin C, vitamin E, bioflavinoids, selenium, zinc, ginkgo biloba, ginseng, pycnogenol, and aloe vera can help prevent free radical damage and premature ageing of the skin. It is thought that these substances may be more effective for the skin when applied externally than if used internally, because a direct application will not be used elsewhere in the body.

EMOLLIENTS soothe, soften, and protect the skin.

EXFOLIANTS are used to encourage the sloughing off of old, dead skin cells from the surface of the skin.

FREE RADICALS are molecular particles – unstable atoms that have an unpaired electron. When trying to stabilize, they steal another atom's electron. As the first becomes stabilized, the other, then, has an unpaired electron, becoming a free radical...and it continues as a chain reaction. Although the body is capable of handling some free radicals, it can't keep up with the amount that is created in the body by today's environment. Over-exposure to the ultraviolet rays of the sun, infections or disease, physical or mental exhaustion, hormonal imbalance, pollution, alcohol, fatty foods, and cigarette smoke all contribute to the formation of free radicals. Free radicals increase oxidation, damage cells ,and promote disease and ageing. The skin reflects this onslaught of free radical damage in the form of dryness, wrinkling, loss of elasticity, and 'age spots.'

HUMECTANTS are ingredients that attract and hold moisture to the skin. Because moisture plays such an important role in the condition of the skin – keeping it moist and supple, preventing wrinkles, and promoting softness and smoothness – humectants are important ingredients, especially in moisturizers.

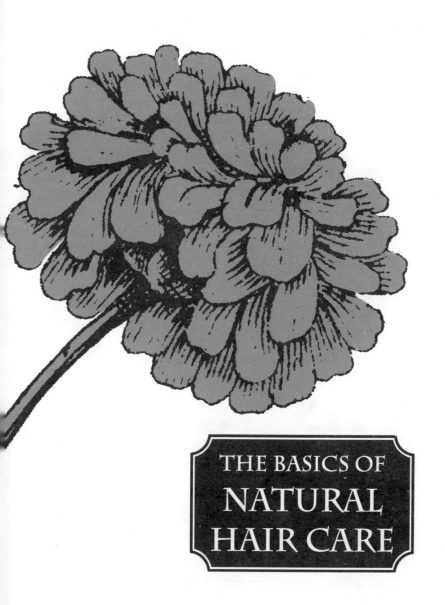

THE BASICS OF
NATURAL
HAIR CARE

DETERMINING YOUR HAIR TYPE

A beautiful, healthy head of hair is an asset to anyone's appearance. A natural hair care program of regular trims, proper brushing, gentle cleansing, and effective conditioning will leave your hair in its most attractive state: moving freely, reflecting light in a spectrum of colors, and expressing your individuality. Knowing your hair type will help you determine which products are best for your hair and how your hair should be treated. In this process, assess the part of the hair shaft that is nearest the scalp.

Normal. Normal hair refers to hair that is benefitting from well-balanced sebaceous glands that are producing just the right amount of oil to keep the hair in good condition. Normal hair is not plagued with chronic split ends or tangling. It appears shiny, has good elasticity, and grows at a healthy rate.

Dry. There are two causes of dry hair. First, the hair will be dry if the sebaceous glands that lubricate the hair shaft are underactive, thus not producing enough oil to protect the hair. Secondly, hair will be dry if it has been damaged in a way that causes both moisture and oil loss. This damage can result from several factors that will be described in this chapter, such as chemical treatments or heat. Dry hair has a dull appearance, poor elasticity, and split ends.

Oily. Oily hair is the result of over-active sebaceous glands. Though oily hair is usually in good condition because of the abundance of oil, it is a condition that causes other problems. It does not have the light, clean, fluffy appearance that people desire, and often oily hair causes skin problems around the hair line. Oily hair is usually frequently shampooed, which can leave the ends dry or damaged while the scalp area appears oily.

Another consideration in determining your hair type is the size of the diameter of the hair shaft, generally catagorized as fine, medium, or coarse. If you have fine hair, it needs to be handled gently because it will become dry and damaged more easily than the other types. Medium hair has an average strength and coarse hair is the strongest. The strength of the hair determines how much mistreatment it can withstand before becoming damaged.

THE NATURAL HAIR CARE PROGRAM

I was once asked to teach a class entitled "Nutritional Influences on the Hair and Skin" to a group of young women in a cosmetology school. Visually scanning my audience, I had their ages pegged between twenty-five and thirty on the basis of their appearances. To my surprise, I later found out that this was a group of high school seniors – about seventeen years old! In trying to understand what had thrown off my judgment, I realized it was the dull, lack-luster appearance of permed, over-processed hair (typical of cosmetology students). It is not uncommon for young women of this age to want to look older. However, when women begin to age and want to recapture a youthful appearance, a shiny, healthy head of hair can do just that! (The condition of the skin is the first factor in a woman's appearance that will age her, and the condition of her hair is the second.)

Physiologically, the hair on the top of your head may have been designed to keep your head warm and help to hold in body heat. However, today, for all practical purposes, it is an adornment. It is used as an avenue of self-expression and to project a certain image of character – as unique and individual as the people themselves.

There is an average of 100,000 hairs growing on a person's head. Hair is composed of a protein called keratin, and because it has no nerves, hair is considered a non-living tissue. A single strand of hair will last anywhere from two to four years and then a new hair will push it out and replace it. It is normal to lose as many as seventy-five hairs a day.

Embedded in the scalp beneath the surface of the skin is a tube-like structure called the hair *follicle*. It is the shape of this follicle that will determine whether the hair will grow straight or curly. In every hair follicle there is a sebaceous gland producing an oil called *sebum* that gives luster, pliability, and protection to each hair strand. At the base of the hair follicle is the *papilla,* which is the hair 'manufacturing plant'. The papilla is fed by the bloodstream, which carries the nourishment to produce a new hair.

Hair has the same simple needs to keep it healthy as any other part of the body: nourish it, nurture it, and do not mistreat it. Following is a natural hair care program that is unsurpassed in improving the health and appearance of the hair as well as eliminating many hair and scalp problems.

STEP #1:
THE HAIRCUT

*T*he foundation and beginning of taking care of your hair is to get an appropriate haircut. Your haircut should be designed to suit your lifestyle, the texture of your hair, the amount of hair you have, the shape of the hair (straight or curly), and the shape of your face. The hair design should be in proportion to your body. A competent hairstylist can help you find a design which works for you as well as flatters your appearance. Whatever the cut, get a trim every couple of months to maintain the hairstyle and give it a finished look. Even people who are letting their hair grow longer will benefit from regular trims by eliminating the ends that are drying out and may be starting to split.

STEP #2:
BRUSHING

*T*he old notion of brushing the hair a hundred strokes a day to keep it healthy and shiny is fine advice if the brushing is done correctly and if the hair is strong enough to handle it. Fine hair that is dry or damaged would do better with fewer strokes. However, once you have determined the number of strokes suitable for your hair, a daily brushing is a good treatment.

Brushing the hair will leave the hair shiny, lint free, and untangled. It increases circulation to the scalp and stimulates hair growth. For the health of the scalp and hair, brushes made with natural bristles or fibers are the best because they absorb the hair's natural oils and spread it down the length of the hair shaft, making the brushing process a conditioning treatment. Because of the texture of the fiber, these brushes do an excellent job of removing minute particles of dust and dirt from the hair without creating static.

The correct procedure for brushing long hair is to begin at the ends, removing any large tangles with your fingers. The hair should be dry. Never brush the hair when it is wet as it is more vulnerable to weakening and breakage. (If you must 'get through' your hair while it is wet, use a large toothed comb or your fingers.) Continue brushing, picking up more hair and working up the length of the hair shaft until you reach the scalp. Then, brush thoroughly from the scalp to the hair ends with long continuous strokes. Shorter hair can usually be brushed from the scalp to the ends right away. For added benefit, bend over at the waist and brush the hair down toward the floor. This is very stimulating. It encourages hair growth by increasing circulation and the flow of vital nutrients to the papilla. It also feels great!

A proper and thorough brushing should precede every shampoo.

STEP #3:
CLEANSING

*T*here are no set rules as to how often to shampoo because everyone's hair is different. Some people wash their hair twice a day – in the morning and again at the end of the day. To the other extreme, I know an elderly woman who washes her hair twice a year (although she rinses it whenever she bathes). Her scalp produces very little oil and her hair has always been very dry, growing drier with age. So, she found it stayed in good condition if she brushed it well everyday and washed it very little. Most of us would fall between these two examples, which serve to illustrate that the frequency of shampooing is a matter of personal preference and need. General guidelines would dictate that oily hair be washed every one or two days and less oily hair might be washed once or twice a week.

Choosing a shampoo is also an individual decision. The action and fragrance will vary with different products. Use the same guidelines as mentioned for skin care to find a quality product (See "A Checklist for Beautiful Skin – # 6). Before you buy, read the labels and choose a product that is formulated for your hair type. Do not purchase products that contain harsh ingredients, artificial colors, and artificial fragrances – they can be irritating, expensive, and unnecessary to the real purpose of shampooing, which is to clean the hair and scalp. In addition, artificial colors and fragrances are common allergens and should be avoided.

Well-formulated shampoos will contain gentle cleansing agents (the most common is sodium laureth sulfate), plant oils, herbal extracts and true essential oils. Essential oils of rosemary and lavender are especially good for the hair. Rosemary has been used as a hair tonic for hundreds of years. It is an anti-dandruff treatment, it is believed to stimulate hair growth, and it is an excellent conditioner. Lavender has a balancing effect as a scalp treatment, and it is a good hair conditioner that leaves a lovely scent. Special ingredients such as aloe vera, jojoba oil, or seaweed are also beneficial. After you have purchased your shampoo and brought it home, dilute it before you use it. This is particularly important if you have long, dry, or damaged hair. In an empty squeeze bottle (or an empty shampoo bottle), put one part shampoo and four parts of water and mix. This is a practice that is done by the finest hair salons. In this dilution, the shampoo is less harsh to the hair and it rinses more thoroughly without leaving a residue. It will clean just as well – although, sometimes, you will not get as much lather.

Before you apply the shampoo to your hair, rinse your hair well with warm (not hot) water. Shampoo should not be applied to dry hair. This first rinsing acts as a pre-wash to remove dust and water-soluble dirt.

Then, apply the diluted shampoo to the scalp area where there is the most oil and massage, covering the entire scalp. Try not to tangle the hair and avoid scrubbing the ends of the hair, particularly if your hair is long. The ends are the oldest and driest part of the hair shaft. Oil from the scalp, the hair's natural conditioner, will not reach the ends of long hair and, therefore, the ends really do not need to be lathered. After this step – rinse, rinse, rinse with water. Shampoo that is not thoroughly rinsed from the hair leaves a residue that can dry the hair, attract dirt, and irritate the scalp. If you shampoo everyday, lather only once, even if you have oily hair. Over-cleansing can create a 'vicious cycle' of stimulating oil production and drying out the hair. If you shampoo less frequently, experiment with one or two latherings. If you are satisfied with the results of just one, stick to that. It is better for the hair.

STEP #4:
PH-BALANCED RINSE

*A*fter a thorough shampooing and water rinsing, follow with an acid pH rinse. This is a million dollar beauty treatment for only pennies. It removes detergent or soap residue left from the shampooing process, promoting cleaner and shinier hair. It conditions and soothes the scalp and replaces the protective acid mantle on the scalp and the hair shaft. It is also a measure for preventing dandruff. To prepare, pour two tablespoons of apple cider vinegar in three cups of warm water and stir. Pour slowly through the hair and massage well into the scalp for about one minute. Follow with a thorough rinsing of clear water. At this point, some people like to change the water temperature from warm to cool. The cool water is very refreshing and exhilarating and is said to make the hair shinier.

STEP #5:
CONDITIONING

*C*onditioning is not necessary for everyone nor is it necessary to condition the entire head of hair. This step should be tailored to the needs of the hair. Those with short hair in good condition may not need a conditioner at all. People with long hair may need to apply the conditioner only to the ends where the hair is lacking natural oils. Permed, colored, high-lighted, or otherwise chemically treated hair should be completely conditioned on a regular basis.

There are a variety of commercial conditioners available of varying qualities. As with shampoo, avoid those with artificial colors and fragrances. Natural food stores have excellent products, conscientiously made without harmful ingredients or animal testing. Look for conditioners that contain true essential oils and plant oils. Castor oil is a natural hair strengthener and is excellent in hair conditioning formulas.

Conditioning treatments become necessary for the hair when it has been damaged. Because hair is not a living tissue, it cannot repair itself. Though conditioning treatments can help restore luster and vitality to the hair, prevention is the best cure. Hair is damaged externally by heat (natural and unnatural), chemicals, over-manipulation, or a combination of these three. The symptoms of damaged hair are excessive tangling, split ends, breakage, a dull appearance, and poor elasticity (a healthy strand of hair can be stretched a little without breaking).

AVOID THE HAIR DESTROYERS: HEAT, CHEMICALS, AND OVER-MANIPULATION

HEAT

*D*ry heat damages the hair by disrupting the moisture balance. The following is a list of heat 'culprits' with suggestions for counteracting their damaging effects:

- **Blow dryers.** Allow your hair to air dry. When that is

not possible, use the blow dryer to simulate a warm wind. Use a low temperature setting and keep it moving – do not concentrate in one spot. I suggest leaving a small amount of moisture in the hair – an amount that will quickly air dry. This way, you will be sure you have not over-dried your hair.

- **Hot rollers.** They cause split, dry ends and breakage. To minimize the damage, use only a high quality set that has been designed to be gentle on the hair. Use end papers for extra protection. Try not to use hot rollers everyday – twice a week at most.

- **Curling irons.** These harm the hair in the same way hot rollers do but have more of a tendency to burn the ends. Do not use a curling iron unless you have strong, healthy hair. For long hair, there is a way to use a curling iron so that the ends are rolled in last. Ask your hair stylist to demonstrate this for you. Also, be certain your hair is completely dry before using the iron or the set will not hold and you will have to curl it again.

- **The sun.** Ah, the wonderful, life-giving sun...how it wreaks havoc with our skin and hair! If you spend long hours in the sun, protect it with a hat or bandana, especially if your hair has been chemically treated.

CHEMICALS

Chemicals are the second category of offenders and are probably the worst culprits for lifeless hair. Harsh chemicals are everywhere and often inescapable. There is chlorine in the tap water, pollutants in the air, and many poor quality commercial cosmetic products on the market. Common beauty salon services can also cause chemical damage to the hair. Permanent wave solutions are made of strong chemicals that cause the hair to become dry and lose its shine – especially after repeated applications. Constant conditioning is required to help replenish the hair. Hair 'dyeing' or 'tinting' and bleaching services damage the hair in much the same way that permanents do. The cuticle of the hair shaft is raised which causes oil and moisture loss, getting worse with repeated applications. Bleaching leaves the hair especially dry and brittle. Also, be aware that hair care products such as styling mousse, hair spray, or gels can contain harmful, irritating ingredients.

OVER-MANIPULATION

Over-manipulation refers to mechanical damage to the hair. Pulling the hair too tightly in rubber bands or too tightly around curlers can cause hair damage and breakage. Barrettes that are too tight can break the hair. Brushing the hair when it is wet is another form of over-manipulation that is harmful. "Traction baldness" can be caused by over-manipulation and results from pulling the hair, with tension, in the same direction over a long period of time. This will tend to discourage growth, particularly around the hairline. I have seen this in young children whose hair has been pulled back tightly in a pony-tail over a long period of time.

It is not uncommon for hair to be subjected to a combination of these three hair destroyers: heat, chemicals, and over-manipulation. If this is the case for your hair, plenty of conditioning and gentle care are required. Try to eliminate one or more of the culprits.

INTERNAL HEALTH

A final consideration for the health of the hair concerns the internal health of the individual. Anne Marie Colbin, author of <u>Food and Healing</u>, has observed dramatic changes in the hair of her students after they switch to a whole foods diet. As the new hair grows in, Colbin says, "One can actually see the change in diet and health chronicled in the hair shaft." There are several important dietary influences on the hair. Protein can have a dramatic effect on texture – too little results in dry hair that grows slowly. A diet low in the fatty acids found in oils can cause thin and dry hair in as little as two to three months. The best oils to include in your diet are olive, canola, or avocado. Foods rich in vitamin A are also critical. "A deficiency <u>or</u> excess of this nutrient can cause hair loss," says Charles Rudy, clinical nutritionist. You can also supplement your diet with food rich in biotin, a powerful vitamin for hair growth. Biotin is found in most beans, fish, and whole grains, especially brown rice. Anything that stimulates circulation stimulates hair growth, so regular exercise is important.

All the physical, mental, and emotional factors that contribute to good health will also affect the hair. However, most hair that is not looking its best is caused from external damage and improper care.

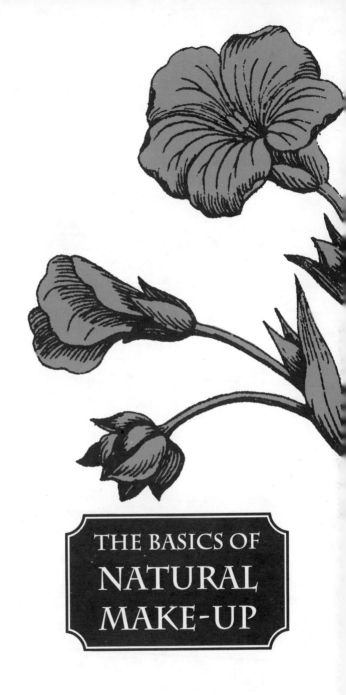

THE BASICS OF
NATURAL
MAKE-UP

MAKE-UP ARTISTRY

*M*ake-up artistry is the use of design and color to accentuate the best features of our faces and minimize the poor ones. This accentuation can liven or 'perk up' our appearance, making us look more youthful, and has definite psychological benefits for helping us feel that we 'look our best.'

Make-up artistry requires make-up products, an understanding of color and design, and experience in application.

MAKE-UP PRODUCTS

- **CONCEALER** is used to cover skin discolorations and blemishes and to even skin tone in specific areas. Typically, it is used for dark circles under the eyes, blemishes, and 'age spots.'

- **FOUNDATION** is designed to even skin tone with coverage that matches the natural complexion color. It is available in sheer (minimal coverage) to opaque (maximum coverage). It is not necessary to use foundation all over the face – use it only where it is needed or desired. Blend the foundation at the jawline. It is not recommended to apply foundation on the neck because it will rub off on clothing. Be aware that the color of your foundation may need to change with the season, particularly if you are exposed to the sun. Never try to change the color of your natural skin tone with a foundation. It will look very artificial and mask-like.

- **TRANSLUCENT POWDER** is used to set make-up so it will last longer and to create a smooth, even, velvety finish. It helps to prevent shine-through of oily skin and helps to minimize color and texture imperfections. Translucent powder is best applied with a large fluff brush. It is excellent when used in the T-zone of combination skin to cut down the shine.

- **EYESHADOW** is used to enhance the appearance of the eyes through color and design. It is applied on the eye lid and upper eye lid as well as under the lower lashes. Eye shadow powders can be applied with a damp sponge applicator for a more intense color. Powder eyeshadows are less likely to crease than cream shadows.

- **EYELINER (EYE PENCIL)** was initially designed to make the lashes look thicker. Today they are also used to accentuate, define, and design the shape of the eye. The best way to sharpen eyelining pencils is to put them in the freezer overnight. In the morning, sharpen as usual.

- **MASCARA** is used to define, thicken, and lengthen the natural lashes.

- **BLUSHER** is used to 'perk up' the complexion and create a youthful look. It is applied to the cheeks and is considered to be the #1 beauty booster. A blusher unifies or 'pulls together' the appearance of the face.

- **LIP PENCIL AND LIPSTICK** are used to define and emphasize the lips.

THE APPLICATION

*B*egin a make-up application on a clean face that has been moisturized. The make-up will last longer if the moisturizer has been allowed to set for ten to twenty minutes. If this is not possible, apply the moisturizer sparingly.

Make-up can be applied in whatever order suits you, but generally it is applied in this sequence: concealer, foundation, translucent powder, eye liner, eye shadow, mascara, blush, lip liner, and lipstick.

A NINE-STEP MAKE-UP APPLICATION

1. **Apply concealer** (cover stick) to any area of discoloration that you would like to hide. If you need to apply a thick layer of concealer, use two light applications rather than one heavy one. Do not apply concealer on 'crow's feet' at the corner of the eye. Instead, apply moisturizer.

2. **Apply foundation** using a make-up sponge or your fingertips, blending quickly. Foundation blends much better when the skin has been properly moisturized. The two most common mistakes made with foundation are using the wrong color and using too much.

3. **Apply translucent powder** with a large fluff brush in downward strokes over the face – the direction the hair grows. Generally, translucent powder is not applied

around the eyes – particularly on mature skin. Very dry or wrinkled skin should use translucent powder sparingly because it can make the skin look drier.

4. **Brush the eyebrows** into shape. First, brush all the hairs straight up, and then sweep them to the side. If you need to add color to your eyebrows, use a brow pencil in short, natural-looking strokes. Follow with brushing, which will blend and soften the color.

5. **Apply eye shadow** with a light touch, adding more if needed. As a general rule, when using three colors, put the lightest on the brow bone, the medium on the lid and the darkest in the crease. Be aware that too much eye shadow can make the eyes look smaller. If you use several different colors, be certain to blend them well and make sure that they look attractive when the eye is looking downward.

6. **Apply eye liner (eye pencil)** in a design that flatters the shape of your eyes. The eyeliner is applied very close to the lashes – even in between the lashes. It can be applied completely around the eye, just on the upper lid, just on the lower lid, on half of the upper and half of the lower, or any variation that is flattering or serves the purpose of your design. Try a variety of designs, such as just a 'v' of liner in the outer corner. If you apply liner on the lower lid, 'set' it with a little powder eye shadow – it will last longer.

7. **Apply mascara** sparingly, one coat at a time. Apply one coat to the upper and lower lashes. Allow to dry completely between coats. Repeat, if desired. If clumping occurs, use a brush or eyelash comb to separate the lashes. Eyelashes can be powdered with translucent powder between coats for extra thickness. Comb or brush the eyelashes between coats to avoid caking or clumping.

8. **Apply blusher** sparingly with a fluff brush. Blend the blusher perfectly onto the cheeks where you would naturally blush. This area is called the apple of the cheek. Do not apply too near the nose or too far out on the cheek. If you are over thirty-five, use blusher sparingly. At this age, just a hint of color looks the most natural. If you have applied too much, cover over it with your translucent powder.

9. **Outline the lips,** using a lip pencil. Although lip lining can be used to subtly change the shape of your lips, it must be done carefully to avoid an unnatural look. Once the lips have been lined, **use the lipstick** to fill in. Blot. For long-lasting lip color, moisturize the lips, apply foundation and translucent powder, then apply lipcolor and blot.

USING COLOR IN MAKE-UP ARTISTRY

*C*olor is defined as the quality of an object or substance with respect to the light that is reflected by it. The key word in this definition is 'light.' Without light, there is no color. Each of the colors in a full spectrum is a vibration that travels in waves, each having a different length. Red is the longest and violet is the shortest. From these colors, the color wheel was invented. A color wheel has primary colors, which are red, blue, and yellow, and the secondary colors, which are orange, green, and purple. Next, there are the intermediary colors which include every color in between the primaries and secondaries, and the combinations are infinite. It is from this color wheel that all colors are possible. Neither white nor black is considered a color.

The color wheel is divided into colors that are 'cool' and colors that are 'warm.' The warm colors have more yellow in them and the cool colors have more blue in them.

Understanding color can help us to use it more artistically in make-up application. Using it well creates a masterpiece and using it poorly can mean an aesthetic disaster. When selecting the colors for your make-up, notice the given set of personal colors with which you have to work – the color of your eyes, your hair, and your skin. The colors you choose for make-up should complement these natural colors.

UNDERSTANDING COLOR

Colors are never isolated or seen by themselves. They are usually next to another color. It is this relationship of colors that will make them 'work' (please the eye) or 'not work.' Comparing and moving colors around is very helpful in understanding individual colors and how they work together.

Color and its relationships are subjective. Not only do people physically perceive color slightly differently, but they also feel differently about different colors. What is beautiful to one person may not be to another.

If the use of color is subjective, then there are no rules for its use. If there are no rules, how do you pick colors for a make-up application? By experience and guidelines. It is your experience that will make you a make-up artist. Using guidelines is always safe but may lack flair and personal expression. However, guidelines are great for getting started until your experience can dictate your choice and use of color.

GENERAL GUIDELINES FOR MAKE-UP COLOR SELECTION

*A*pplying make-up can be one of the most creative and fun expressions of the artist within us all. It can transform plain women into gorgeous creatures. There are two main factors to consider before applying make-up:

- *What colors are you going to use?*
- *What design (the placement of color) are you going to use?*

To determine what colors to use, first look at yourself in the mirror without any make-up. What color are your eyes, your skin, and your hair? Are they warm or cool colors? Remember that warm has yellow undertones and cool has blue undertones. If you are uncertain, look at the palms of your hands and see if they have more yellow or more blue. If you are still uncertain, compare your palms with other peoples' palms. This is an example of the relationship of color. If you have three palms to compare, you will see how different skin tones can be and which ones look more yellow or more blue.

Generally, you will want to use warm-color make-up on warm-colored skin. The same is true for cool-colored skin. Don't forget to use contrasting colors in the same family by using light and dark of the same shade.

Before you begin applying the make-up, be clear in your mind what it is you are trying to achieve. An excellent way to get started with this is to collect pictures from magazines, especially make-up advertisements, that show a make-up application that you like. You can pick from these to practice on yourself. Select make-up application pictures that are on women that have coloring similar to yours.

COLOR GUIDELINES FOR MAKE-UP PRODUCTS

CONCEALERS are available in neutral tones, usually light, medium, and dark. Use a concealer that is only one or two shades lighter than your natural skin coloring. If it is too light, it will draw attention to the area.

FOUNDATIONS come in a range of warm, neutral, or cool colored bases. Choose a color that most closely matches your natural skin tone and remember that colors look darker in the bottle than they do on the skin. Foundations can be mixed together for a customized blend. Test for correct color selection on your jawline, not on your hand or wrist. Select the color in natural light.

TRANSLUCENT POWDERS are available in light, medium, and dark shades. Choose a shade that most closely matches your foundation.

EYESHADOWS are available in a wide range of colors and should be selected on the basis of the color of the eyes, the skin tone, the hair color, and the clothing that is going to be worn. Choose colors that will contrast and enhance your natural eye color, such as brown shadow for blue eyes. Do not match your natural eye color with your eyeshadow color. If the color of your eyes is light, use a light touch in applying shadow – so it is not overpowering.

Try these suggested colors:

> **Blue eyes:** browns, copper, smoky charcoal, plum, pinks, greens
>
> **Green eyes:** rusty browns, copper, apricot, navy blues, pinks, plum, teal
>
> **Brown eyes:** blue-grey, olive green, forest green, plum, violet, contrasting shades of brown
>
> **Grey eyes:** silver, beige, lighter blues, teal.
>
> **Hazel eyes:** muted greens, muted blues, muted turquoise, plum

EYELINERS are available in many colors but the most often used are black, brown, grey, blue, and green. Generally, black is good for dark-eyed brunettes. Brown is used for blondes, brunettes, and redheads. Grey is good for people with 'cool' skin tones. Blue looks very good on people with blue or grey eyes. Green is used on redheads and green-eyed people.

MASCARA comes in a selection of colors with the most popular being black, brown, grey, and blue. The color of the mascara should compliment the color of the eyes. Matching the eyeliner with the mascara will create the illusion of very thick lashes.

BLUSHER color selection depends on the skin tone. Warm skin tones should use warm-colored blushers such as peaches and corals. Cool skin tones should use cool-colored blushers such as pinks, roses, or plums. Darker complexions can wear brighter colors. Lighter complexions should wear softer, more subtle colors. The blusher and the lipstick color should be from the same color group though they can be of different intensities.

LIP PENCILS AND LIPSTICKS are available in many colors. The color selection depends on the skin tone – warm or cool. Other considerations are the color of the eyes, the hair, and the clothes that are to be worn. The lip pencil should match either the color of your lips or the color of your lipstick. Avoid frosts if you have very full lips. Avoid very dark colors if your lips are small.

USING NATURALLY PIGMENTED COSMETICS

*U*nfortunately, most of the color cosmetics that are found in the marketplace use artificial FD&C (Food, Drug & Cosmetic) colors in their formulas, especially lipsticks, foundations, and blushers. The use of artificial colors has had a controversial history. In 1900, when they first appeared in manufacturing, there were no regulations governing their use.

The same dyes for clothes could be used for food or cosmetics. Legislation to control the use of artificial colors began in 1906 and continues today, and a list of colors considered safe for use has been established. When problems arise, colors may be removed from the list. This occurred in 1950, when children became ill from specific oranges and reds, and in 1976, one of the most commonly used colors, FD&C Red #2 was de-listed because it was found to cause tumors in laboratory animals.

The controversy exists because almost all artificial FD&C colors approved for use by the Federal Drug Administration are made from coal tar oil or are synthetically produced from petroleum products. These derivatives have been shown to cause cancer when injected into the skin of mice. Yet, despite these findings, they are still used in the manufacturing of food and cosmetics. Why?

The FDA says that the risk is small and may only pose a problem in sensitive people. Even when the FDA recommends the de-listing of a suspicious color, it comes up against vigorous resistence and political pressure from the industry and the manufacturers. Established regulations take time and plenty of public concern to be revoked. The wheels of change turn too slowly, if ever, and the responsibility of guarding our health falls to ourselves.

The negative aspects of using artificial colors are far-reaching. Not only are they a concern for human health but also for the health of the environment and animals. In humans, these substances are suspected carcinogens. In addition, empirical evidence has proven them to be sensitizers that can cause allergic responses. In the 1960's, innovative studies were conducted by Benjamin Feingold, M.D., who made the connection between artificial colors and behavior and learning problems in children. Today, the Feingold Association, a non-profit organization for the chemically sensitive, estimates that one in ten people is affected. Symptoms of this sensitivity may include headaches, nausea, lack of concentration, life-threatening asthma attacks, fatigue, irritability, nervousness, and confusion. Jane Hersey, the director of the Feingold Association, states, "Artificial colors and other synthetic chemicals can affect us whether we ingest them, breathe them, or just come in contact with them with our skin (which can absorb small amounts)." If this is the case, women are subjecting themselves to unnecessary risks. Not only is make-up worn on the skin where particles can be inhaled or absorbed, lipstick is worn on the mouth, where, surely, small amounts are ingested. So, even though make-up is worn externally, it can affect us internally.

Another hazard that must be considered is the impact of artificial colors on the environment. If they pose potential health risks, then we certainly do not want them floating around in our air and water. While it is possible to avoid them in cosmetics, if we so choose, we cannot avoid them in our food and water chain, and, if they are in the food and water chain, we must consider how these can affect plants, animals, and the delicate balance of ecosystems.

USING NATURALLY PIGMENTED COSMETICS

There are real manufacturing difficulties in using natural pigments. Working with them is more time consuming, especially in the developmental and formulating stages. These pigments can behave inconsistently and can have unexpected results. Sometimes the coloring strength of one batch will be stronger or weaker than the last, so each batch has to be color matched with the desired original shade.

Natural pigments can come from annatto (yellow-orange), fruit juice and vegetable juice concentrates (a variety of colors), grape skin extract (red-purple), beet powder (deep purple), beta carotene (yellow-orange), turmeric (yellow to golden brown), carmine (dark pink), paprika (red-orange), and caramel (dark brown). Iron oxides are used from the mineral world and provide a whole range of blues, greens, and violets, and titanium dioxide is used to produce white.

Natural pigments are far more expensive than artificial colors. A natural color may cost $200.00 a pound while it may cost as little as $20.00 a pound for the artificial counterpart. In addition, to achieve the desired shade, more of the natural pigment is frequently needed because the coloring ability is not as powerful as the synthetics. Another disadvantage is that there is a limited range of colors, so some desirable cosmetic colors are not possible to obtain from nature.

Despite these manufacturing hurdles, a few dedicated and visionary manufacturers have persevered and have made available lipsticks, eyeshadows, blushers, mascaras, and eye-liner pencils using natural colors. These are not inferior products in which the consumer must settle for less in order to live more healthfully. No, these are full lines of beautiful, classic colors that are tastefully packaged, reasonably priced, and longlasting.

For those of you who have not yet tried naturally pigmented make-up, you will be delightfully surprised to see how attractively the colors blend and harmonize with the natural color tones of your skin, hair, and eyes. There is no need to compromise your standards. If you are committed to having a healthy lifestyle, then the time is right to commit yourself to healthy make-up.

BIBLIOGRAPHY

Modern Esthetics: A Scientific Source for Estheticians
by Henry J. Gambino. Milady Publishing Co. 1992.

Advanced Professional Skin Care
by Peter T. Pugliese, M.D. APSC Publishing 1991.

The Complete Book of Essential Oils & Aromatherapy
by Valerie Ann Worwood. New World Library 1991.

Aromatherapy: An A-Z by Patricia Davis.
Saffron Walden. The C.W. Daniel Company Limited 1988.

The Smoker's Book of Health
by Tom Ferguson. Putnam & Sons 1987.

The Principles of Holistic Skin Therapy with Herbal Essences
by Dietrich Gumbel. Karl F. Haug Publishers 1986.

Whole Body Healing
by Carl Lowe,. James W. Nechas. Rodale Press 1983.

Dr. Braly's Optimum Health Program
by James Braly, M.D. Times Books 1985.

Food and Healing
by Annemarie Colbin. Ballantine Books 1986.

Healthy Healing by Linda G. Rector-Page, N.D., Ph. D.
Healthy Healing Publications 1992.

A Consumer's Dictionary of Cosmetic Ingredients
by Ruth Winter. Crown Publishers 1989.

Hands by Linda Rose. The Overlook Press 1980.

The Herbal Handbook
by David Hoffman. Healing Arts Press 1988.

The Art of Breathing by Nancy Zi. Bantam Books 1986.

The Complete Book of Water Therapy
by Dian Dincin Buchman. E.P. Dutton 1979.

Diet for Natural Beauty
by Aveline Kushi. Japan Publications 1991.